Ketogenic Breakfast Recipes

A Collection of Salty and Sweet Keto Recipes for a Healthy Breakfast

By Carla Wilson

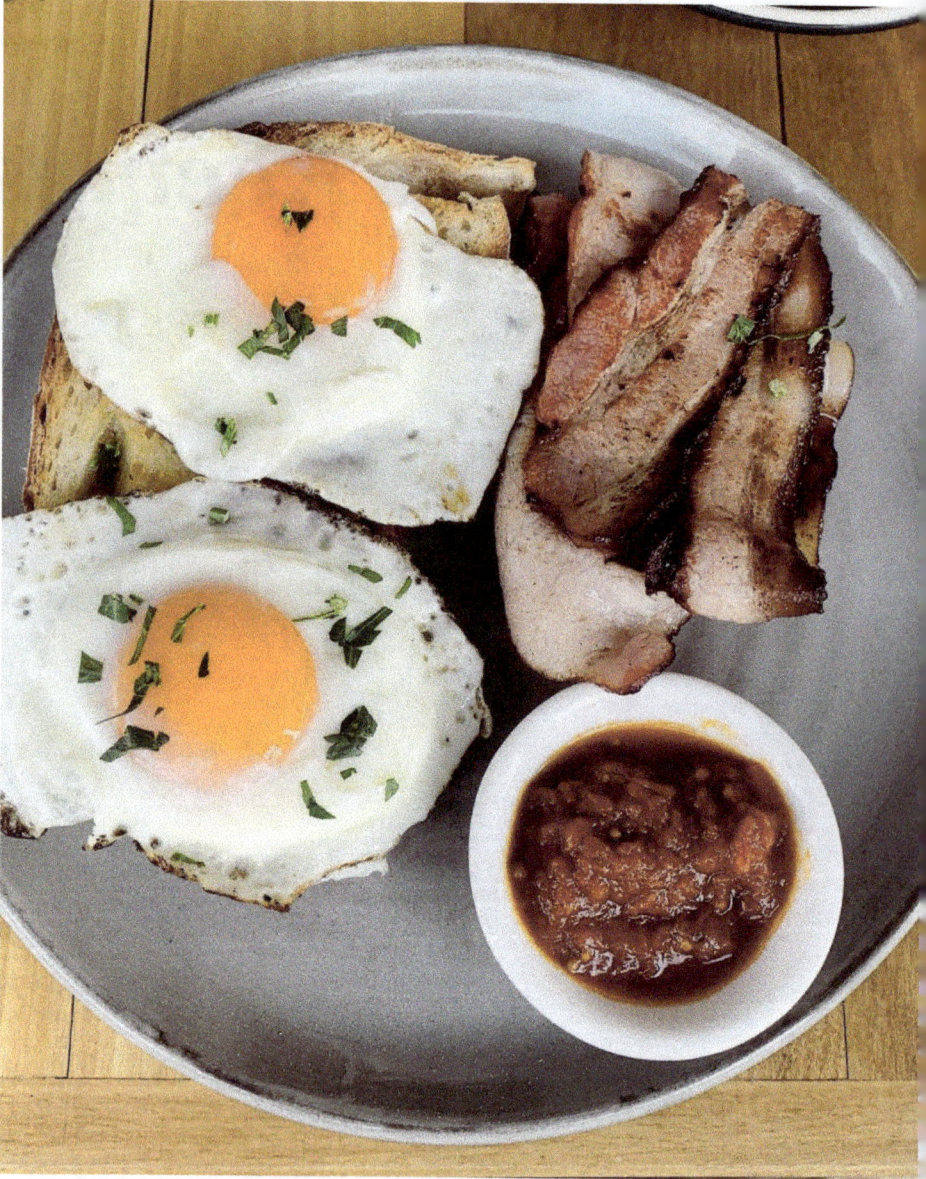

content within this book has been derived from various sources. Please consult a licensed professional before attempting any techniques outlined in this book.

By reading this document, the reader agrees that under no circumstances is the author responsible for any losses, direct or indirect, which are incurred as a result of the use of information contained within this document, including, but not limited to, — errors, omissions, or inaccuracies.

Table of Contents

Scrambled Eggs with Mushrooms and Cheese..............10

Peanut Butter Chocolate Smoothie.....................11

Cream Cheese Pancakes 13

Coconut Chia Pudding................................14

Morning Hash 15

Spanish Scramble....................................17

Cheese Waffles 18

Spinach Frittata 19

Keto Oatmeal..21

Baked Eggs 22

Blueberry Smoothie 24

Quick Keto Pancakes 25

Spinach Quiche 27

Cream Crepes 29

Smoothie Bowl 31

Almond Butter Muffins...............................33

Classic Western Omelet..............................35

Sheet Pan Omelet....................................37

Detoxifying Green Smoothie 38

Nutty Pumpkin Smoothie..................................40

Kale Wrapped Eggs.......................................41

Zucchini Keto Bread 43

Ham Sausage Quiche......................................46

Coconut Almond Breakfast................................48

Avocado Egg Muffins.....................................51

Soft-Boiled Eggs..53

Breakfast Casserole.....................................56

Poblano Cheese Frittata.................................59

Poached Egg 62

Spinach Egg Bites.......................................64

Bacon Cheeseburger Waffles 67

Keto Breakfast Cheesecake...............................71

Egg-Crust Pizza 73

Breakfast Roll-Ups......................................75

Basic Opie Rolls 77

Almond Coconut Egg Wraps 79

Bacon & Avocado Omelet 80

Bacon & Cheese Frittata 82

Bacon & Egg Breakfast Muffins...........................83

Bacon Hash 86

Keto Peanut Butter Bars 87

Keto Chocolate Crunch Bars..89

Keto Coconut Chocolate Bars 91

Keto Lemon Bars...93

Chocolate Chip Pumpkin Protein Bar 96

Keto Flourless Chocolate Cake 98

Brownie Cheese Cake... 100

Peanut Butter Molten Lava Cake 102

Chocolate Japanese Cheesecake.................................... 104

Italian Cream Cake 106

Scrambled Eggs with Mushrooms and Cheese

Preparation Time: 10 minutes

Cooking Time: 20 minutes

Serving: 4

Ingredients:

- 4 tablespoons butter
- 8 eggs
- 4 tablespoons Parmesan cheese, shredded
- Salt and black pepper, to taste
- 1 cup fresh mushrooms, chopped finely

Directions:

1. Mix together eggs, salt, and black pepper in a bowl and beat well. Melt butter in a non-stick pan and add the beaten eggs. Cook for about 5 minutes and add Parmesan cheese and mushrooms. Cook for another 5 minutes, stirring occasionally. Let cool slightly and enjoy

Nutrition:

- 203 Calories
- 17.5g Fats
- 11.2g Proteins

Peanut Butter Chocolate Smoothie

Preparation Time: 5 minutes

Cooking Time: 0 minutes

Serving: 1

Ingredients:

- 1 tablespoon unsweetened cocoa powder
- 1 cup unsweetened coconut milk
- 1 tablespoon unsweetened peanut butter
- 1 pinch sea salt
- 5 drops stevia

Directions:

1. 1Mix all the ingredients until smooth. Pour into a glass and serve immediately.

Nutrition:

- 79 Calories
- 5.7g Fats
- 3.6g Proteins

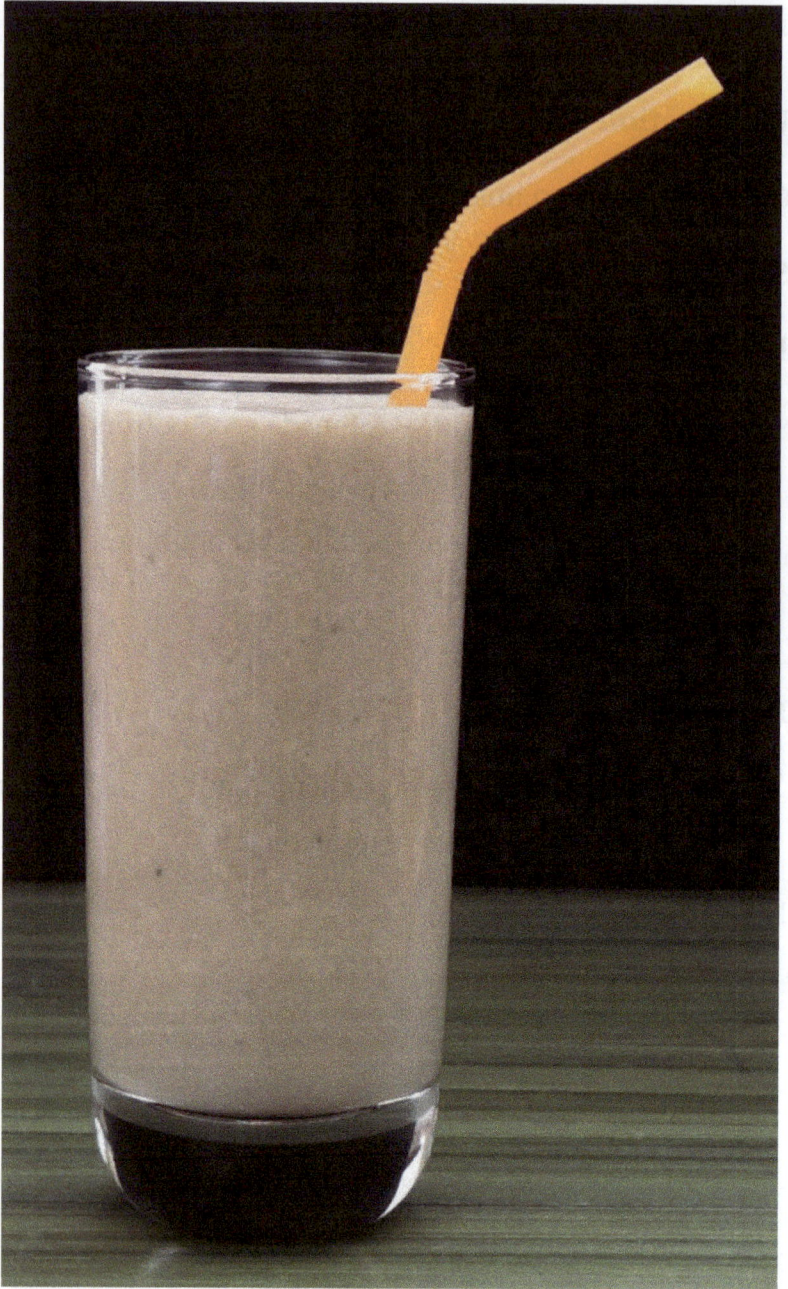

Cream Cheese Pancakes

Preparation Time: 5 minutes

Cooking Time: 12 minutes Serving: 4

Ingredients:

- 2 eggs
- ½ teaspoon cinnamon
- 2 oz. cream cheese
- 1 teaspoon granulated sugar substitute
- ½ cup almond flour

Directions:

1. Mix all the ingredients until smooth. Transfer the mixture into a medium bowl and put aside for about 3 minutes. Grease a large non-stick skillet with butter and add ¼ of mixture. Spread the mixture and cook until golden brown. Flip the pancake and let it cook. Do it again for the remaining mixture.

Nutrition:

- 170 Calories
- 4.3g Carbs
- 14.3g Fats
- 6.9g Proteins

Coconut Chia Pudding

Preparation Time: 10 minutes

Cooking Time: 25 minutes

Serving: 4

Ingredients:

- 1 cup full-fat coconut milk
- ¼ cup chia seeds
- ½ tablespoon honey
- 2 tablespoons almonds
- ¼ cup raspberries

Directions:

1. Mix together coconut milk, chia seeds, and honey in a bowl and refrigerate overnight.

Nutrition:

- 158 Calories
- 6.5g Carbs
- 14.1g Fats
- 2g Proteins

Morning Hash

Preparation Time: 10 minutes

Cooking Time: 30 minutes

Serving: 2

Ingredients:

- ½ teaspoon dried thyme, crushed
- ½ small onion, chopped
- 1 tablespoon butter
- ½ cup cauliflower florets, boiled
- ¼ cup heavy cream
- Salt and black pepper, to taste
- ½ pound cooked turkey meat, chopped

Directions:

1. Finely chop cauliflowers. Sauté butter and onion. Then add chopped cauliflower. Put turkey and let it cook. Mix in heavy cream and keep mixing it. Then serve.

Nutrition:

- 309 Calories
- 3.6g Carbs
- 34.3g Protein
- 17.1g Fat

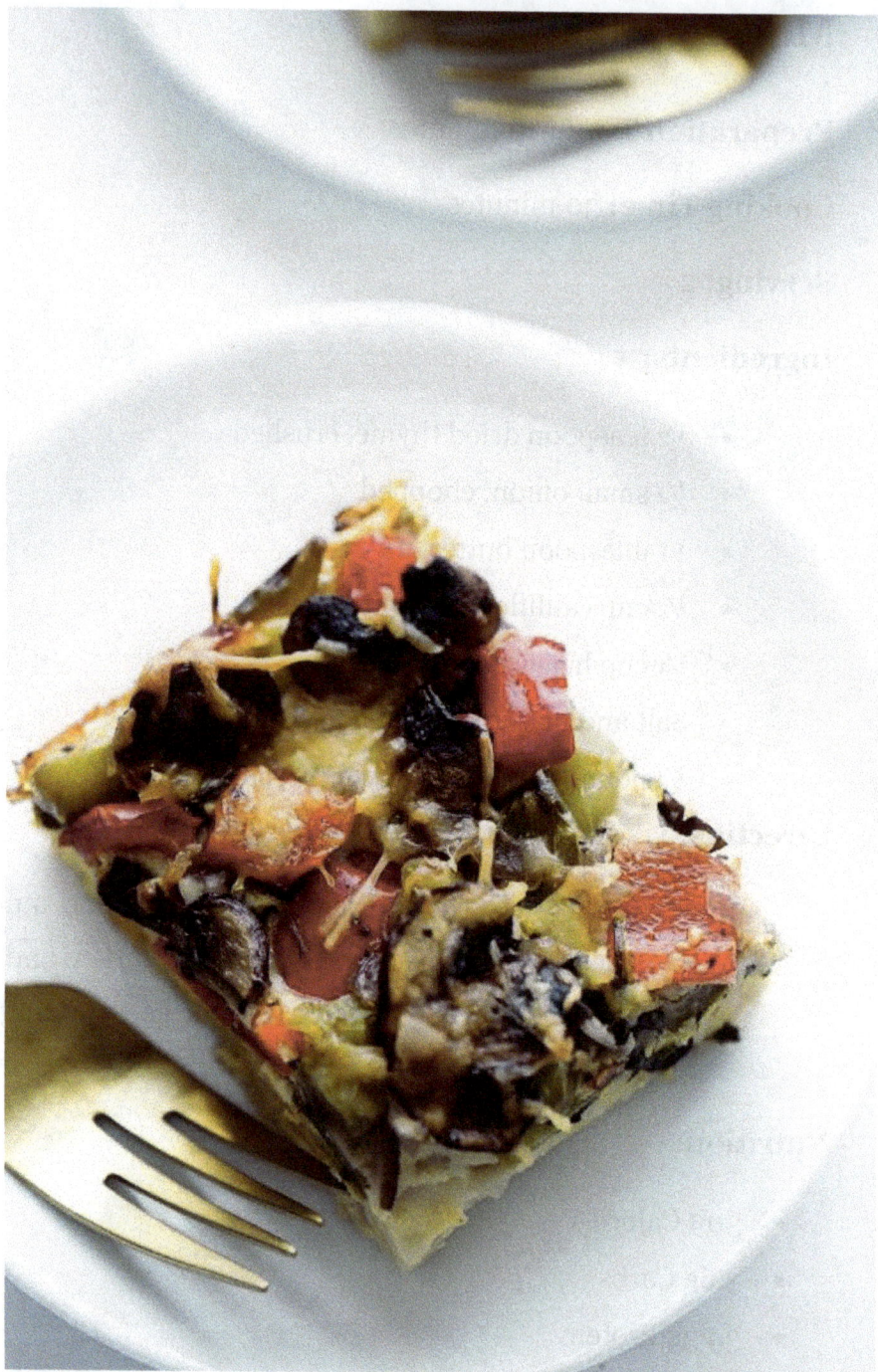

Spanish Scramble

Preparation Time: 10 minutes

Cooking Time: 20 minutes

Serving: 2

Ingredients:

- 3 tablespoons butter
- 2 tablespoons scallions, sliced thinly
- 4 large organic eggs
- 1 Serrano chili pepper
- ¼ cup heavy cream
- 2 tablespoons cilantro, chopped finely
- 1 small tomato, chopped
- Salt and black pepper, to taste

Directions:

1. Mix cream, eggs, cilantro, salt and black pepper in a bowl. Sauté butter, tomatoes and Serrano pepper. Then add egg mixture and let it cook. Immediately serve it and topped with scallions

Nutrition:

- 180 Calories
- 2g Carbs
- 6.8g Protein

- 16.5g Fat

Cheese Waffles

Preparation Time: 10 minutes

Cooking Time: 20 minutes

Serving: 2

Ingredients:

- ½ cup Parmesan cheese, shredded
- 2 organic eggs, beaten
- 1 teaspoon onion powder
- 1 cup mozzarella cheese, shredded
- 1 tablespoon chives, minced
- ½ teaspoon ground black pepper
- 1 cup cauliflower
- 1 teaspoon garlic powder

Directions:

1. Mix all ingredients. Grease a waffle iron and heat it. Cook the mixture by batch until golden brown. Serve.

Nutrition:

- 149 Calories
- 6.1gCarbs
- 13.3g Protein
- 8.5g Fat

Spinach Frittata

Preparation Time: 20 minutes

Cooking Time: 45 minutes

Serving: 2

Ingredients:

- 1½ ounce dried bacon
- 2 ounces spinach, fresh
- 1½ ounce shredded cheese
- ½ tablespoon butter
- ¼ cup heavy whipped cream
- 2 eggs
- Salt and black pepper, to taste

Directions:

1. Grease and preheat oven at 360 degrees. Heat butter in a skillet and add bacon. Cook until crispy and add spinach. Stir thoroughly and keep aside. Mix eggs and cream. Then transfer it to the baking dish.
2. Add bacon spinach mixture to the baking dish and transfer to the oven. Bake for about 30 minutes and remove from the oven to serve.

Nutrition:

- 592 Calories

- 3.9g Carbs
- 39.1g Protein
- 46.7g Fat

Keto Oatmeal

Preparation Time: 10 minutes

Cooking Time: 20 minutes

Serving: 2

Ingredients:

- 2 tablespoons flaxseeds
- 2 tablespoons sunflower seeds
- 2 cups coconut milk
- 2 tablespoons chia seeds
- 2 pinches of salt

Directions:

1. Mix all ingredients in a sauce pan. Let it simmer. Dish out in a bowl and serve warm.

Nutrition:

- 337 Calories
- 7.8g Carbs
- 4.9g Protein
- 32.6g Fat

Baked Eggs

Preparation Time: 5 minutes

Cooking Time: 10 minutes

Serving: 2

Ingredients:

- 2 eggs
- 3 ounces ground beef, cooked
- 2 ounces cheddar cheese, shredded

Directions:

1. Grease and preheat oven at 390 degrees. Arrange the cooked ground beef in a baking dish. Make two holes in the ground beef and crack eggs in them. Top with cheddar cheese and transfer the baking dish in the oven. Let it bake for 20 minutes. Allow it to cool for a bit and serve to enjoy. For meal prepping, you can refrigerate these baked eggs for about 2 days wrapped in a foil.

Nutrition:

- 512 Calories
- 1.4g Carbs
- 51g Protein
- 32.8g Fat

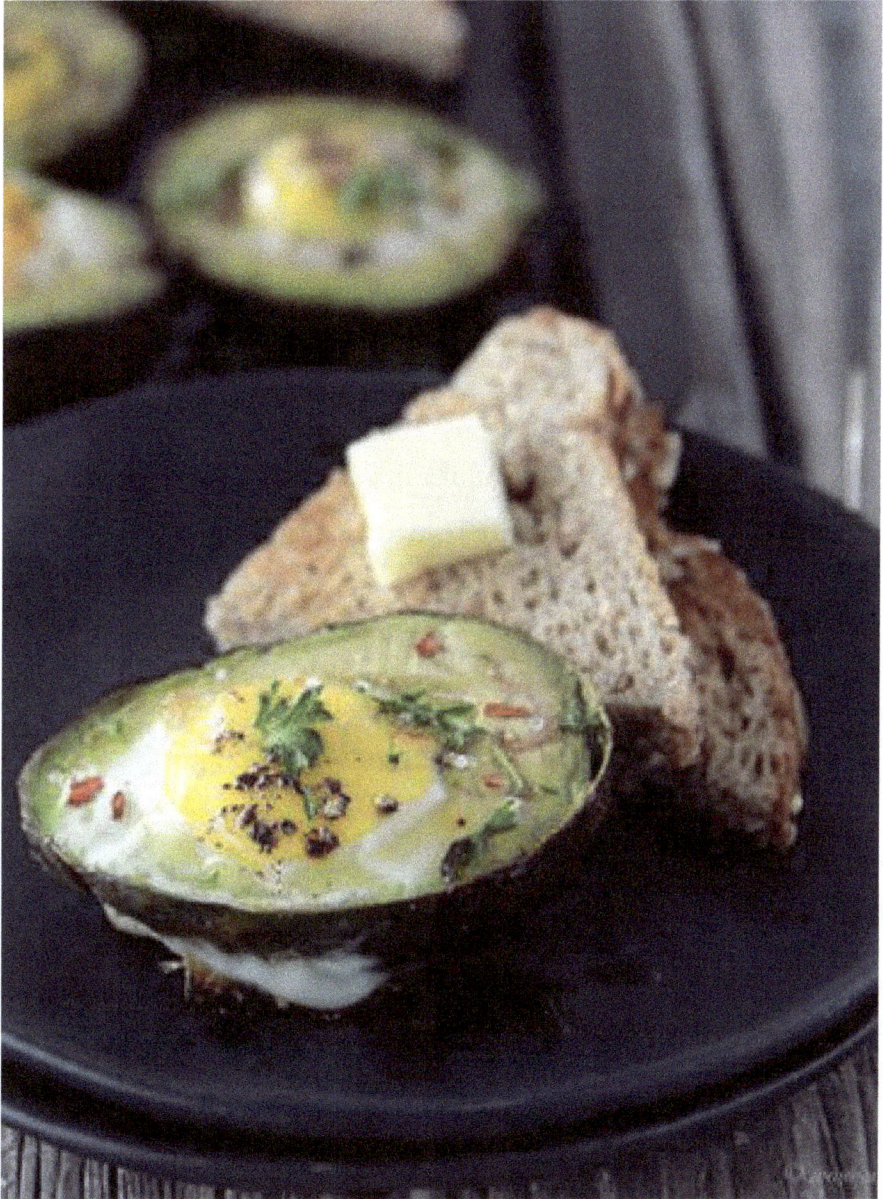

Blueberry Smoothie

Preparation Time: 5 minutes

Cooking Time: 15 minutes

Serving: 2

Ingredients:

- 1 cup fresh blueberries
- 1 teaspoon vanilla extract
- 28 ounces coconut milk
- **2 tablespoons lemon juice**

Directions:

1. Blend all ingredients until smooth. Pour it in the glasses to serve and enjoy.

Nutrition:

- 152 Calories
- 6.9g Carbs
- 1.5g Protein
- 13.1g Fat

Quick Keto Pancakes

Preparation Time: 15 minutes

Cooking Time: 30 minutes

Serving: 2

Ingredients:

- 3 ounces cottage cheese
- 2 eggs
- ½ tablespoon psyllium husk powder, ground
- ½ cup whipped cream
- 1 oz. butter

Directions:

1. Mix all ingredients except whipped cream and keep aside. Heat butter in the frying pan and pour half of the mixture. Cook it on each side and dish out in a serving platter. Add whipped cream in another bowl and whisk until smooth. Top the pancakes with whipped cream on them.
2. Meal Prep Tip: These keto pancakes can also be used as a snack. They taste awesome when serve cold.

Nutrition:

- 298 Calories
- 4.8g Carbs

- 12.2g Protein
- 26g Fat

Spinach Quiche

Preparation Time: 15 minutes

Cooking Time: 30 minutes

Serving: 2

Ingredients:

- 1½ cups Monterey Jack cheese, shredded
- ½ tablespoon butter, melted
- 5-ounce frozen spinach, thawed
- Salt and black pepper
- 2 eggs, beaten

Directions:

1. Grease and preheat the oven to 350 degrees. Heat butter on medium-low heat in a large skillet and add spinach. Cook for about 3 minutes and set aside. Mix together Monterey Jack cheese, eggs, spinach, salt and black pepper in a bowl.
2. Transfer the mixture into prepared pie dish and place in the oven. Bake for about 30 minutes serve by cutting into equal sized wedges.

Nutrition:

- 349 Calories
- 3.2g Carbs

- 23g Protein
- 27.8g Fat

Cream Crepes

Preparation Time: 15 minutes

Cooking Time: 25 minutes

Serving: 2

Ingredients:

- 1 teaspoon Splenda
- 2 tablespoons coconut flour
- 2 tablespoons coconut oil, melted and divided
- 2 organic eggs
- ½ cup heavy cream

Directions:

1. Put 1 tablespoon of coconut oil, eggs, Splenda and salt in a bowl and beat until well combined. Sift in the coconut flour slowly and beat constantly. Stir in the heavy cream and continuously beat until the mixture is well combined.

2. Put half mixture in a pan. Cook each side and repeat with the remaining mixture. Dish out to scrve and enjoy. For meal prepping, wrap each cream crepe into wax paper pieces and place into a resealable bag. Freeze for up to 3 days and remove from the freezer. Microwave for about 2 minutes to serve.

Nutrition:

- 298 Calories
- 8g Carbs
- 7g Protein
- 27.1g Fat

Smoothie Bowl

Preparation Time: 5 minutes

Cooking Time: 0 minutes

Serving: 2

Ingredients:

- ¼ cup unsweetened almond milk
- 1 cup frozen strawberries
- ½ cup fat-free plain Greek yogurt
- 1 tablespoon walnuts, chopped
- ½ tablespoon unsweetened whey protein powder

Directions:

Blend strawberries until smooth. Add almond milk, Greek yogurt and whey protein powder in the blender and pulse for about 2 minutes. Transfer the mixture evenly into 2 bowls and top with walnuts to serve. You can wrap the bowls with plastic wrap and refrigerate for 2 days for meal prepping.

Nutrition:

- 71 Calories
- 19g Fat
- 6.3g Carbs
- 6.8g Protein

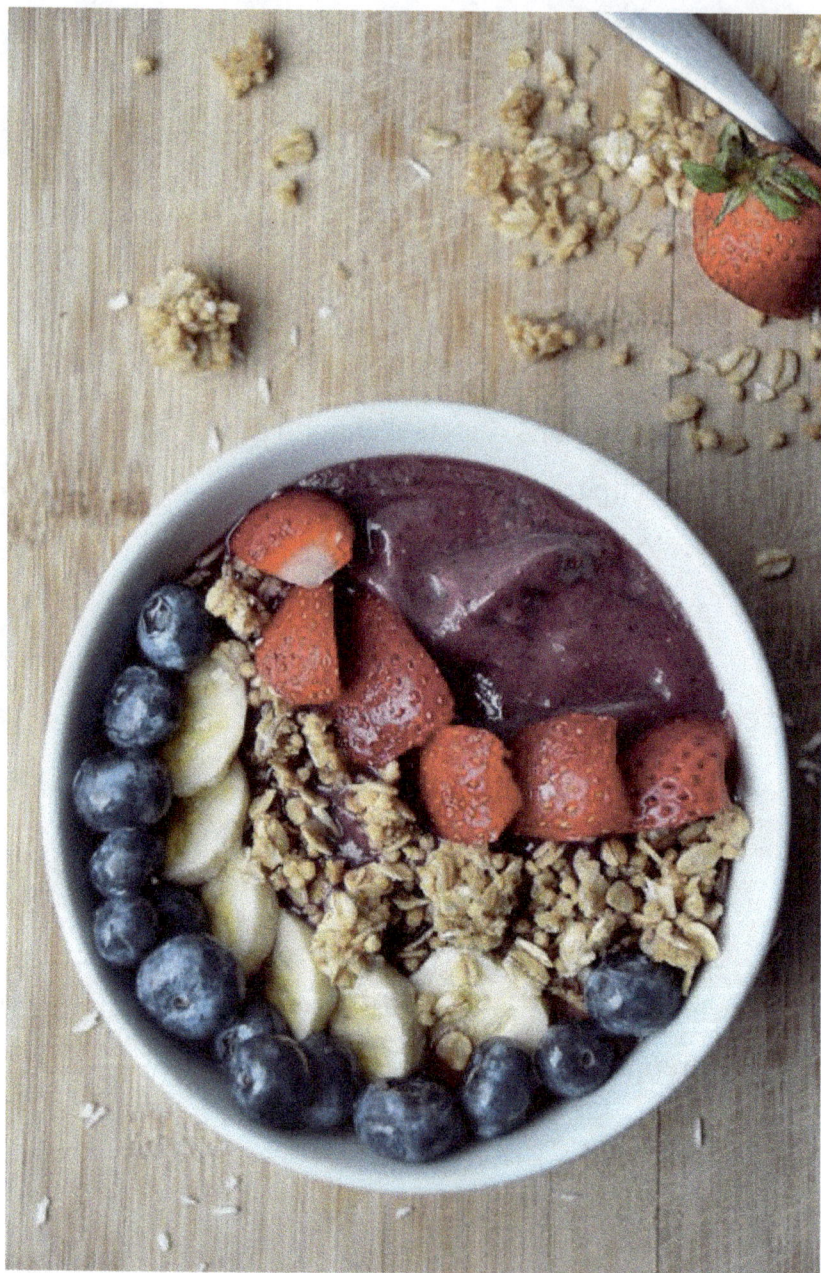

Almond Butter Muffins

Preparation Time: 10 minutes

Cooking Time: 25 minutes

Servings: 6

Ingredients:

- 1cups almond flour
- 1/2 cup powdered erythritol
- 1 teaspoons baking powder
- ¼ teaspoon salt
- ¾ cup almond butter, warmed
- ¾ cup unsweetened almond milk
- 2 large eggs

Directions:

1. Prepare oven to 350 ° F, and line a paper liner muffin pan.
2. In a mixing bowl, whisk the almond flour and the erythritol, baking powder, and salt.
3. Whisk the almond milk, almond butter, and the eggs together in a separate bowl.
4. Fill in wet ingredients into the dry until just mixed together.

5. Spoon the batter into the prepared pan and bake for 22 to 25 minutes until clean comes out the knife inserted in the middle.
6. Cook the muffins in the pan for 5 minutes. Then, switch onto a cooling rack with wire.

Nutrition:

- 135 Calories
- 11g Fat
- 6g Protein

Classic Western Omelet

Preparation Time: 5 minutes

Cooking Time: 10 minutes

Servings: 1

Ingredients:

- 2 teaspoons coconut oil
- 3 large eggs, whisked
- 1 tablespoon heavy cream
- Salt and pepper
- ¼ cup diced green pepper
- ¼ cup diced yellow onion
- ¼ cup diced ham

Directions:

1. Scourge eggs, heavy cream, salt, and pepper.
2. Heat up 1 teaspoon of coconut oil over medium heat in a small skillet.
3. Add the peppers and onions, then sauté the ham for 3 to 4 minutes.
4. Spoon the mixture in a cup, and heat the skillet with the remaining oil.
5. Mix in the whisked eggs and cook until the egg's bottom begins to set.

6. Tilt the pan and cook until almost set to spread the egg.
7. Spoon the ham and veggie mixture over half of the omelet and turn over.
8. Let cook the omelet until the eggs are set and then serve hot.

Nutrition:

- 415 Calories5
- 32.5g Fat
- 25g Protein

Sheet Pan Omelet

Preparation Time: 5 minutes

Cooking Time: 15 minutes

Servings: 6

Ingredients:

- 12 large eggs
- Salt and pepper
- 2 cups diced ham
- 1 cup shredded pepper jack cheese

Directions:

1. Prepare oven to 350°F and grease a rimmed baking sheet with cooking spray. Whisk the eggs in a mixing bowl then add salt and pepper until frothy. Stir in the ham and cheese. Pour the mixture in baking sheets and spread into an even layer. Bake for 13 minutes. Let cool slightly then cut it into squares to **serve.**

Nutrition:

- 235 Calories
- 15g Fat
- 21g Protein

Detoxifying Green Smoothie

Preparation Time: 5 minutes

Cooking Time: 0 minutes

Servings: 1

Ingredients:

- 1 cup fresh chopped kale
- ½ cup fresh baby spinach
- ¼ cup sliced celery
- 1 cup water
- 3 to 4 ice cubes
- 2 tablespoons fresh lemon juice
- 1 tablespoon fresh lime juice
- 1 tablespoon coconut oil
- Liquid stevia extract, to taste

Directions:

1. In a blender, add the broccoli, spinach, and celery. Stir in the rest of ingredients and blend until creamy. Pour into a big glass, and instantly enjoy it.

Nutrition:

- 160 Calories
- 14g Fat
- 2.5g Protein

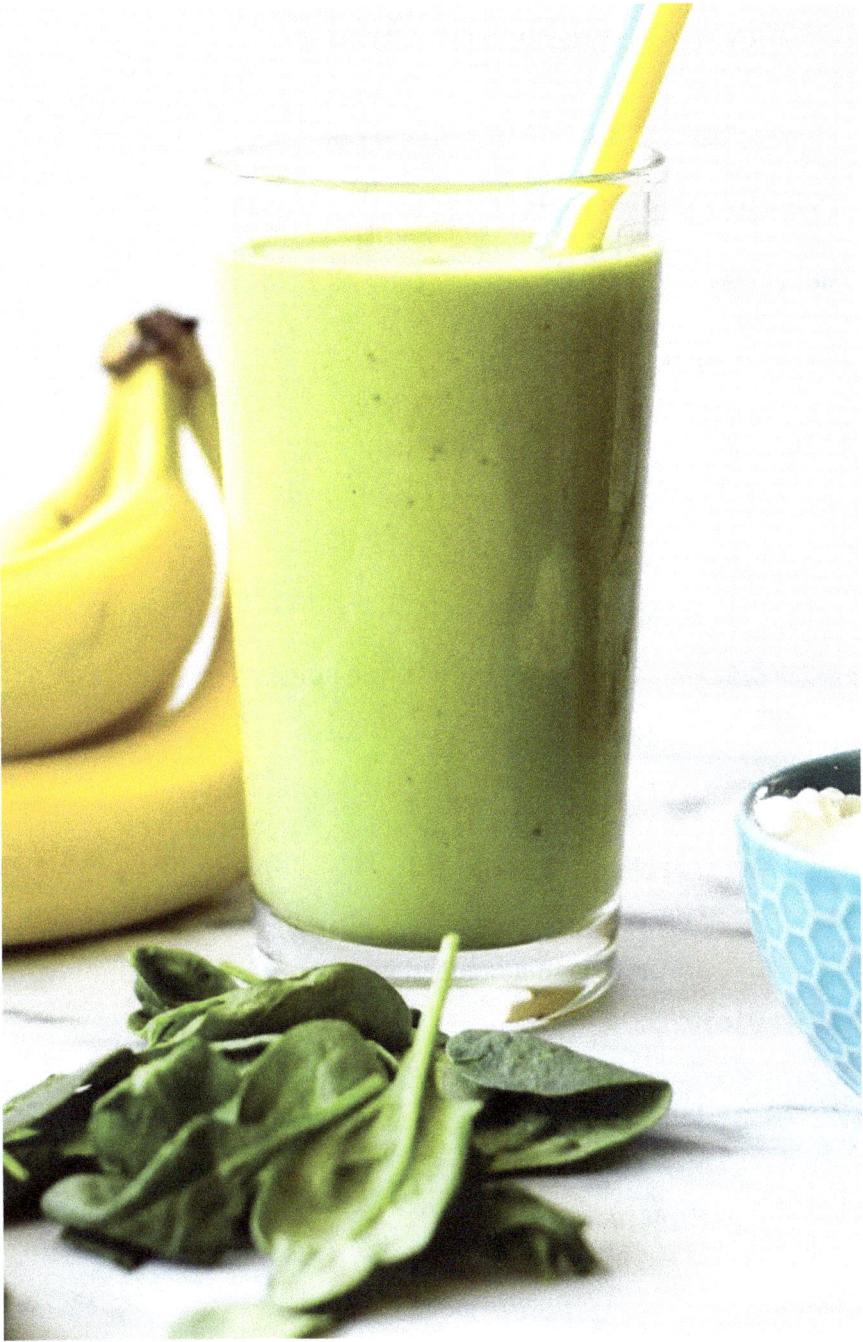

Nutty Pumpkin Smoothie

Preparation Time: 5 minutes

Cooking Time: 0 minutes

Servings: 1

Ingredients:

- 1 cup unsweetened cashew milk
- ½ cup pumpkin puree
- ¼ cup heavy cream
- 1 tablespoon raw almonds
- ¼ teaspoon pumpkin pie spice
- Liquid stevia extract, to taste

Directions:

1. Incorporate all of the ingredients. Pulse the ingredients several times, then blend until creamy. Situate into a large glass and enjoy immediately.

Nutrition:

- 205 Calories
- 16.5g Fat
- 3g Protein

Kale Wrapped Eggs

Preparation Time: 8-10 minutes

Cooking Time: 5 minutes

Servings: 4

Ingredients:

- Three tablespoons heavy cream
- Four hardboiled eggs
- ¼ teaspoon pepper
- Four kale leaves
- Four prosciutto slices
- ¼ teaspoon salt
- 1 ½ cups water

Directions:

1. Peel the eggs and wrap each with the kale. Wrap them in the prosciutto slices and sprinkle with ground black pepper and salt. Place it in your Pressure Pot and pour water. Arrange the eggs over the trivet/basket.

2. Close the lid and lock it. Press "MANUAL" cooking function; timer to 5 minutes with default "HIGH" pressure mode. Allow the pressure to build to cook. After cooking time is over press "CANCEL" setting. Find and press "QPR" cooking function. This setting is for quick release of inside pressure.

3. Slowly open and take it out from the lid.

Nutrition:

- 247 Calories
- 20g Fat
- 19g Protein

Zucchini Keto Bread

Preparation Time: 8-10 minutes

Cooking Time: 40 minutes

Servings: 12-16 slices

Ingredients:

- 1 cup grated zucchini
- 2 ½ cups almond flour
- ½ cup chopped walnuts
- 3 eggs
- ½ cup olive oil
- 1 ½ teaspoon baking powder
- Pinch of ginger powder
- 1 teaspoon vanilla extract
- ½ teaspoon cinnamon
- ¼ teaspoon nutmeg
- pinch of sea salt
- 1 ½ cups water

Directions:

1. Whisk together the wet ingredients in a bowl. Combine the dry ingredients in another bowl. Combine the dry and wet mixture. Stir in the zucchini.
2. Grease a loaf pan and pour the mixture. Top with chopped walnuts. Open its top lid and pour water.

Arrange a trivet or steamer basket inside that came with Pressure Pot. Now arrange the loaf pan over the trivet/basket.

3. Close the lid and press "MANUAL" cooking function; timer to 40 minutes with default "HIGH" pressure mode. Allow the pressure to build to cook the ingredients. After cooking time is over press "CANCEL" setting. Find and press "QPR" cooking function. This setting is for quick release of inside pressure.

4. Slowly open the lid, take out the cooked bread. Cool down, slice, and serve.

Nutrition:

- 164 Calories
- 17g Fat
- 5g Protein

Ham Sausage Quiche

Preparation Time: 8-10 minutes

Cooking Time: 30 minutes

Servings: 4

Ingredients:

- 4 bacon slices, cooked and crumbled
- ½ cup diced ham
- 2 green onions, chopped
- ½ cup full-fat milk
- Six eggs, beaten
- 1 cup ground sausage, cooked
- 1 cup shredded cheddar cheese
- ¼ teaspoon salt
- Pinch of pepper
- 1 ½ cups water

Directions:

1. Grease a baking dish with coconut oil cooking spray. Place all of the ingredients in a bowl, and stir to combine. Add this mixture to the prepared dish.
2. Open its top lid and pour water. Arrange a trivet or steamer basket inside that came with Pressure Pot. Now arrange the dish over the trivet/basket.

3. Close the lid and press "MANUAL" cooking function; timer to 30 minutes with default "HIGH" pressure mode. Allow the pressure to build to cook. After cooking time is over press "CANCEL" setting. Find and press "QPR" cooking function. This setting is for quick release of inside pressure.

4. Place the dish on the rack in your IP and close the lid. Cook on high and release the pressure naturally. Slowly open the lid, take out the cooked recipe in serving plates or serving bowls, and enjoy the keto recipe.

Nutrition:

- 398 Calories
- 31g Fat
- 26g Protein

Coconut Almond Breakfast

Preparation Time: 8-10 minutes

Cooking Time: 5 minutes

Servings: 2

Ingredients:

- 2 tablespoons roasted pepitas
- 1/3 cup coconut milk
- 2 tablespoon chopped almonds
- 1 tablespoon chia seeds
- 1/3 cup water
- One handful blueberries

Directions:

1. Mix the pepitas with almonds and blend well. Switch on the pot. Add the chia seeds with water and coconut milk; gently stir to mix well. Add the pepita mix and combine.

2. Close the lid and press "MANUAL" cooking function; timer to 5 minutes with default "HIGH" pressure mode. Allow the pressure to cook.

3. After cooking time is over press "CANCEL" setting. Find and press "QPR" cooking function. This setting is for quick release of inside pressure. Slowly open and take out the dish from the lid.

Nutrition:

- 148 Calories
- 6g Fat
- 2g Protein

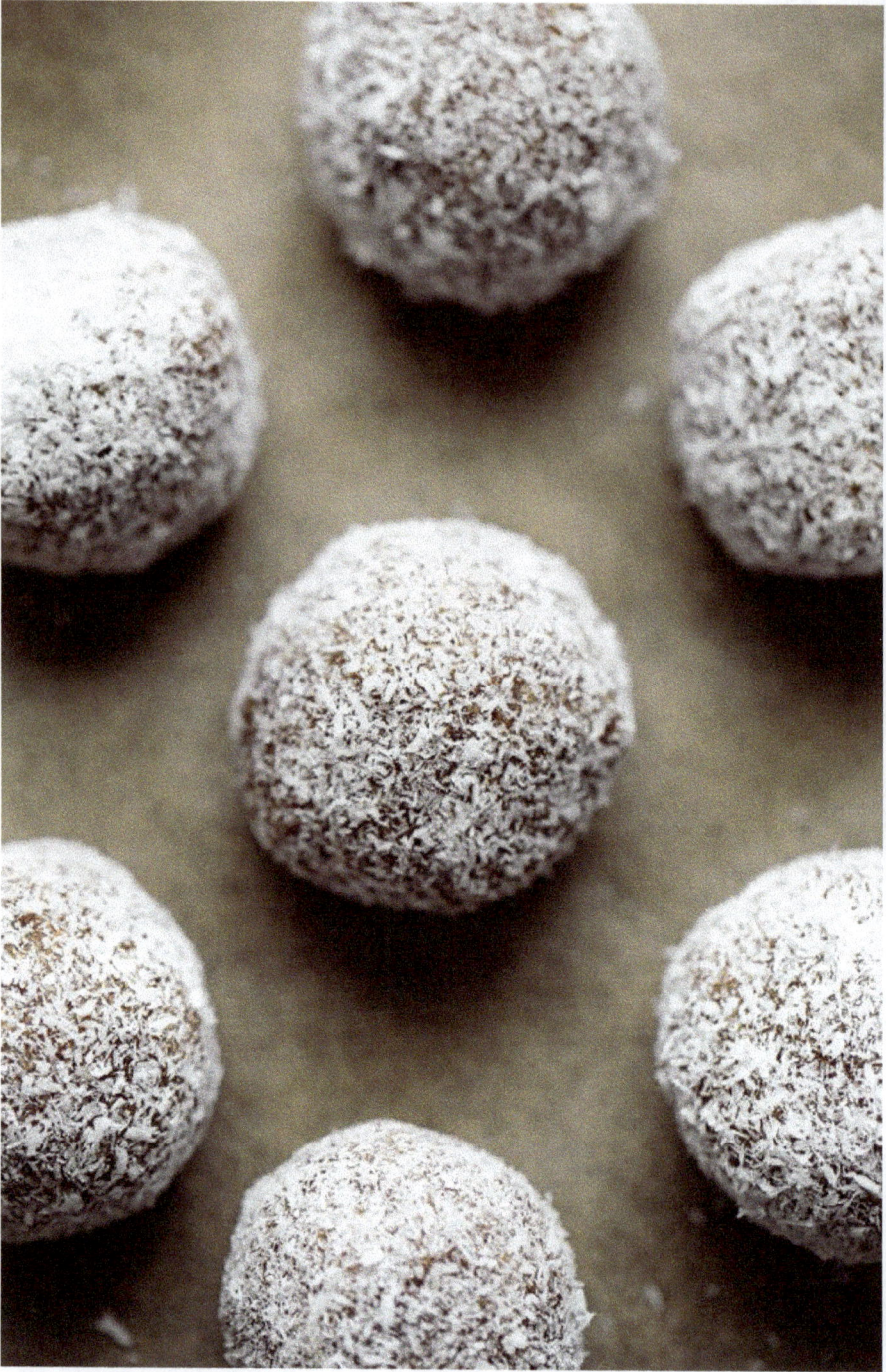

Avocado Egg Muffins

Preparation Time: 8-10 minutes

Cooking Time: 12 minutes

Servings: 4

Ingredients:

- 1 ½ cups of coconut milk
- 2 avocados, diced
- 4 ½ ounces (grated or shredded) cheese
- ½ cup almond flour
- 5 bacon slices, cooked and crumbled
- 5 eggs, beaten
- 2 tablespoon butter
- 3 spring onions, diced
- 1 teaspoon oregano
- ¼ cup flaxseed meal
- 1 ½ tablespoon lemon juice
- 1 teaspoon minced garlic
- 1 teaspoon onion powder
- 1 teaspoon salt
- Pinch of pepper
- 1 teaspoon baking powder
- 1 ½ cups water

Directions:

1. Whisk together the wet ingredients. Stir in the dry ingredients gradually until turns smooth. Stir in the avocado, bacon, onions, and cheese. Add the mixture into 16 muffin cups. Arrange Pressure Pot over a dry platform in your kitchen. Open its top lid and switch it on.

2. In the pot, pour water. Arrange the 8 cups over the trivet/basket.

3. Close the lid and press "MANUAL" cooking function; timer to 12 minutes with default "HIGH" pressure mode. Allow the pressure to cook.

4. After cooking time is over press "CANCEL" setting. Find and press "QPR" cooking function. This setting is for quick release of inside pressure. Slowly open and take out the dish from the pot.

5. Repeat the same process.

Nutrition:

- 146 Calories
- 11g Fat
- 6g Protein

Soft-Boiled Eggs

Preparation Time: 5 minutes

Cooking Time: 3 minutes

Servings: 4

Ingredients:

- 4 Eggs
- 2 cups Water

Directions:

1. Switch on the Pressure Pot, pour in water, insert steamer basket and place eggs in it.
2. Shut the Pressure Pot with its lid in the sealed position, then press the 'manual' button, press '+/-' to set the cooking time to 3 minutes and cook at low-pressure setting; when the pressure builds in the pot, the cooking timer will start.
3. When the Pressure Pot buzzes, press the 'keep warm' button, do a quick pressure release and open the lid.
4. Fill a bowl with ice water, place eggs in it from the Pressure Pot, and let rest for 3 minutes.
5. Then peel the eggs, cut into slices, season with salt and black pepper and serve.

Nutrition:

- 68 Calories4.

- 6g Fat
- 5.5g Protein

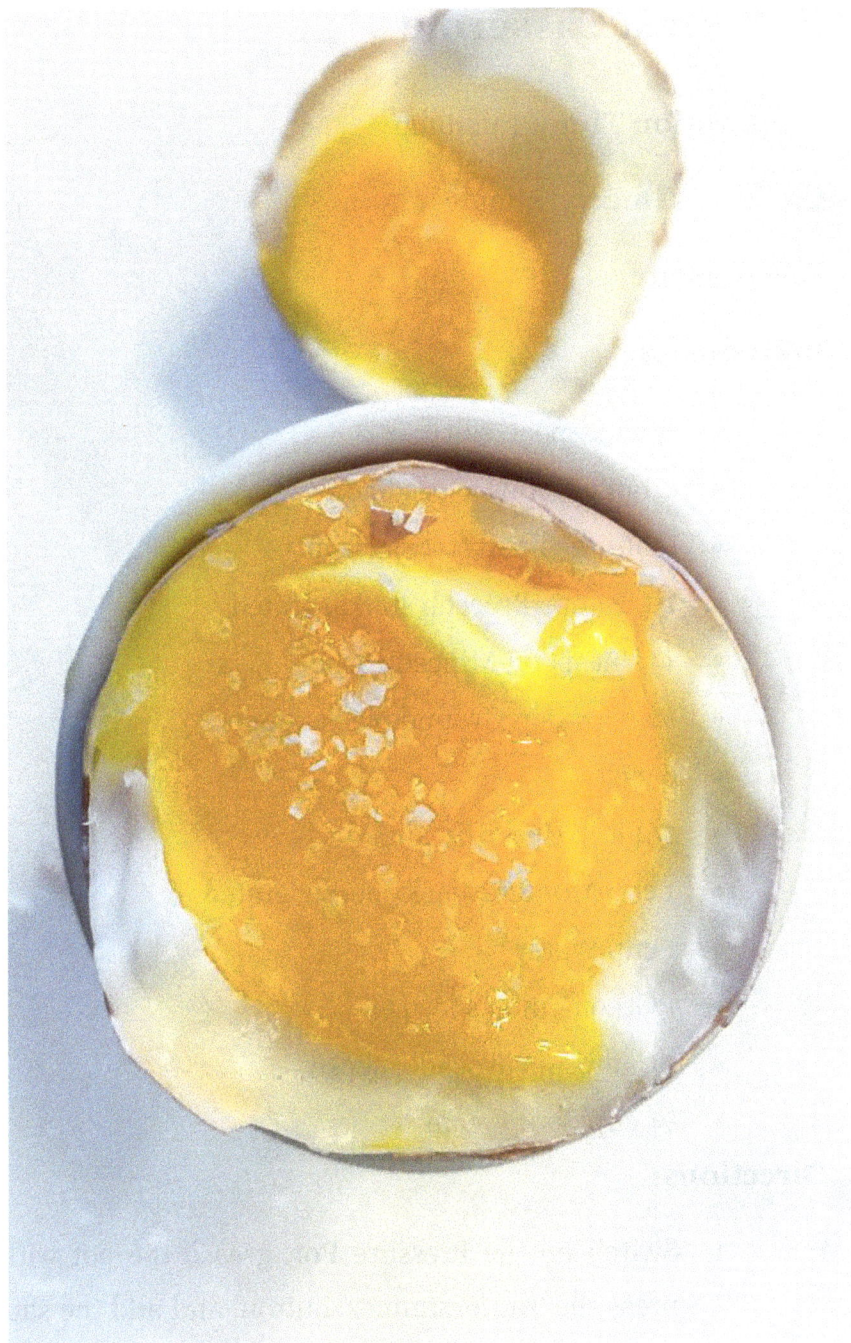

Breakfast Casserole

Preparation Time: 10 minutes

Cooking Time: 45 minutes

Servings: 6

Ingredients:

- 1/2 teaspoon salt
- 2 tablespoons avocado oil
- 6 ounces breakfast sausage
- 1 1/2 cups Broccoli stalks, grated
- 1 tablespoon Minced garlic
- ½ teaspoon Ground black pepper
- 6 eggs
- 1/4 cup Heavy cream
- 1 cup Monterey jack cheese, grated
- 1 cup Water
- 1 Green onion sliced
- 1 California avocado, sliced
- ¼ cup Sour cream

Directions:

1. Switch on the Pressure Pot, grease the pot with oil, press the 'sauté/simmer' button, and add the sausage and cook until the meat is no longer pink.

2. Then add broccoli along with garlic, season with salt and black pepper and continue cooking for 2 minutes.

3. Take a 7-inch baking dish, grease it with oil, spoon in cooked broccoli mixture and spread evenly.

4. Crack the eggs in a bowl, add cream, whisk until combined, and then add onion and cheese, whisk until mixed, pour the mixture over the sausage mixture and cover with aluminum foil.

5. Press the 'keep warm' button, wipe the Pressure Pot clean, pour in water, then insert trivet stand and place baking dish on it.

6. Shut the Pressure Pot with its lid in the sealed position, then press the 'manual' button, press '+/-' to set the cooking time to 35 minutes and cook at high-pressure setting; when the pressure builds in the pot, the cooking timer will start.

7. When the Pressure Pot buzzes, press the 'keep warm' button, release pressure naturally for 10 minutes, then do quick pressure release and open the lid.

8. Take out the baking dish, uncover it and turn it over the plate to take out the frittata.

9. Top the frittata with avocado, cut into slices and the top with sour cream.

Nutrition:

- 351 Calories
- 28.5g Fat

- **18.6g Protein**

Poblano Cheese Frittata

Preparation Time: 5 minutes

Cooking Time: 35 minutes

Servings: 4

Ingredients:

- 4 Eggs
- 10 oz. Diced green chili
- 1 tsp. Salt
- ½ tsp. Ground cumin
- 1 cup Mexican cheese blend, shredded, divided
- ¼ cup Chopped cilantro
- 2 cups Water

Directions:

1. Crack eggs in a bowl, add green chilies, half-and-half, and ½ cup cheese, season with salt and cumin, stir well until incorporated. Take a 6-inch baking dish or silicone pan, grease it with oil, pour in the egg mixture and cover with aluminum foil.

2. Switch on the Pressure Pot, pour water in it, then insert trivet stand and place baking dish on it. Shut the Pressure Pot with its lid in the sealed position, then press the 'manual' button, press '+/-' to set the cooking time to 20 minutes and cook at high-pressure setting;

when the pressure builds in the pot, the cooking timer will start.

3. When the Pressure Pot buzzes, press the 'keep warm' button, release pressure naturally for 10 minutes, then do a quick pressure release and open the lid. Meanwhile, switch on the broiler and let it preheat.

4. Take out the baking dish, spread remaining cheese on top, then place it under the broiler and broil for 5 minutes or until cheese melts and the top is nicely browned.

5. When done, turn the dish over a plate to take out the frittata, then cut into slices and serve.

Nutrition:

- 257 Calories
- 19g Fat
- 14g Protein

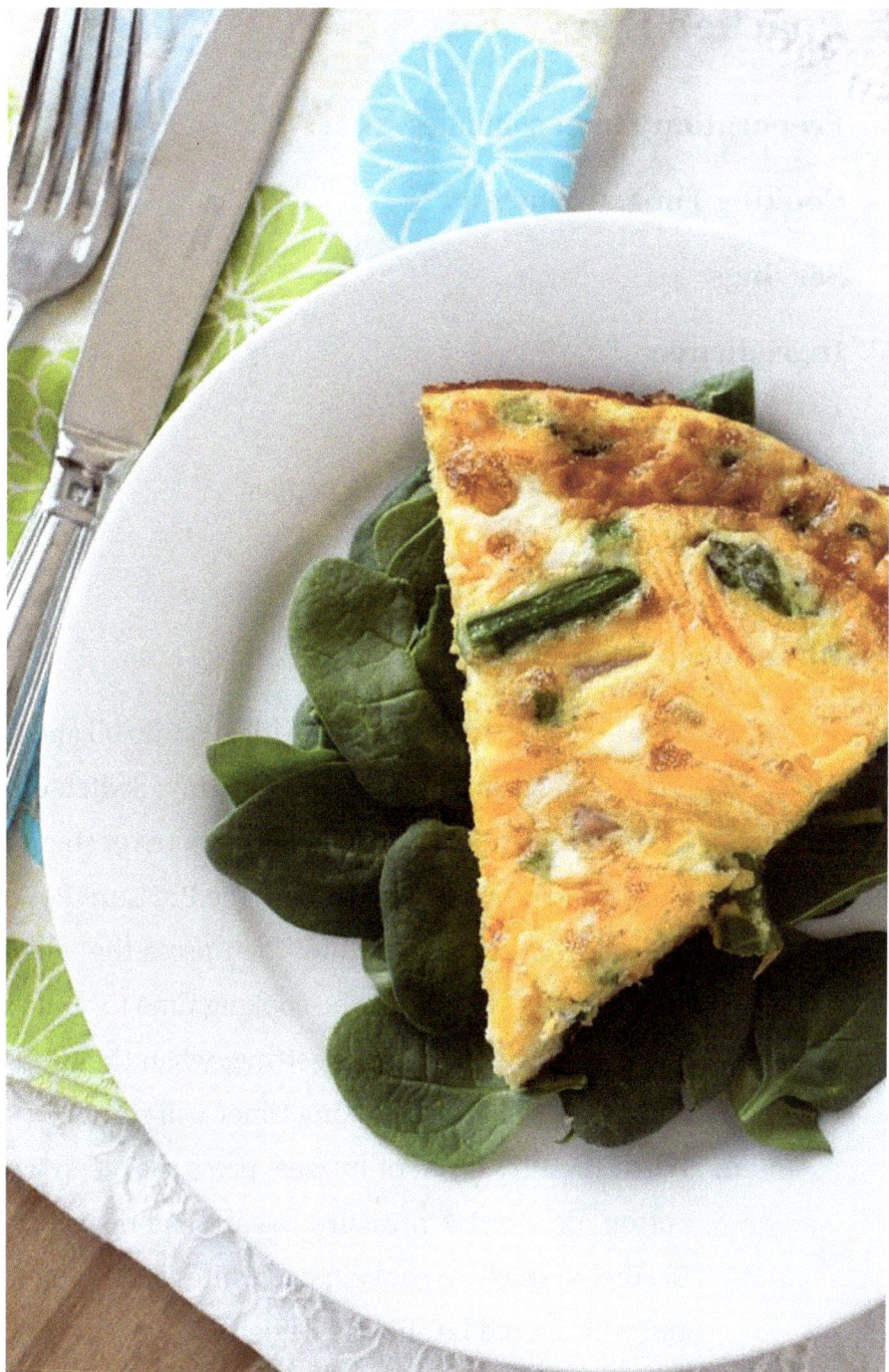

Poached Egg

Preparation Time: 5 minutes

Cooking Time: 7 minutes

Servings: 4

Ingredients:

- ¾ teaspoon salt
- ¾ teaspoon ground black pepper
- 1 cup water
- 4 eggs

Directions:

1. Take a silicone tray, grease it with avocado oil and then crack the eggs into the cups of the tray. Switch on the Pressure Pot, pour water in it, insert a trivet stand and place the silicone tray on it. Shut the Pressure Pot with its lid in the sealed position, then press the 'manual' button, press '+/-' to set the cooking time to 7 minutes and cook at high-pressure setting; when the pressure builds in the pot, the cooking timer will start.

2. When the Pressure Pot buzzes, press the 'keep warm' button, do a quick pressure release and open the lid. Ensure all eggs are cooked; egg whites should be firm, and yolk should be slightly jiggled.

3. Run a knife around each cup in the tray, then gently scoop out the egg and transfer to a serving plate. Season poached eggs with salt and black pepper and serve straight away.

Nutrition:

- 72 Calories
- 4.8g Fat
- 6.3g Protein

Spinach Egg Bites

Preparation Time: 5 minutes

Cooking Time: 20 minutes

Servings: 7

Ingredients:

- 4 Eggs
- ¾ cup Parmesan cheese, grated
- ¼ cup Heavy whipping cream
- ¼ cup Spinach, chopped
- ½ oz. Prosciutto, chopped
- ½ tsp. Ground black pepper
- 1/8 tsp. Salt
- 1 ½ cup Water

Directions:

1. Take an egg bite mold tray having seven cups and fill the cups evenly with prosciutto and spinach. Crack eggs in a bowl, add remaining ingredients except for water and whisk until smooth.

2. Switch on the Pressure Pot, pour in water and place trivet stand in it. Pour egg mixture evenly over spinach and prosciutto, 4 tablespoons per cup or more until 3/4th filled, and then cover the pan with aluminum foil.

3. Place pan on the trivet stand, shut the Pressure Pot with its lid in the sealed position, then press the 'manual' button, press '+/-' to set the cooking time to 10 minutes and cook at high-pressure setting; when the pressure builds in the pot, the cooking timer will start.

4. When the Pressure Pot buzzes, press the 'keep warm' button, release pressure naturally for 10 minutes, then do a quick pressure release and open the lid.

5. Take out the tray, uncover it and turn over the pan onto a plate to take out the egg bites. Serve straight away.

Nutrition:

- 400 Calories
- 29g Fat
- 27g Protein

Bacon Cheeseburger Waffles

Preparation Time: 10 minutes

Cooking Time: 20 minutes

Servings: 4

Ingredients:

Toppings:

- Pepper and Salt to taste
- 12 ounces of cheddar cheese
- 4 tablespoons of sugar-free barbecue sauce
- 4 slices of bacon
- 4 ounces of ground beef, 70% lean meat and 30% fat

Waffle dough:

- Pepper and salt to taste
- 3 tablespoons of parmesan cheese, grated
- 4 tablespoons of almond flour
- ¼ teaspoon of onion powder
- ¼ teaspoon of garlic powder
- 1 cup (125 g) of cauliflower crumbles
- 2 large eggs
- ounces of cheddar cheese

Directions:

1. Shred about 3 ounces of cheddar cheese, then add in cauliflower crumbles in a bowl and put in half of the cheddar cheese.

2. Put into the mixture spices, almond flour, eggs, and parmesan cheese, then mix and put aside for some time.

3. Thinly cut the bacon and cook in a skillet on medium to high heat.

4. After the bacon is cooked partially, put in the beef, cook until the mixture is well done.

5. Then put the excess grease from the bacon mixture into the waffle mixture. Set aside the bacon mix.

6. Use an immersion blender to blend the waffle mix until it becomes a paste, then add into the waffle iron half of the mix and cook until it becomes crispy.

7. Repeat for the remaining waffle mixture.

8. As the waffles cook, add sugar-free barbecue sauce to the ground beef and bacon mixture in the skillet.

9. Then proceed to assemble waffles by topping them with half of the left cheddar cheese and half the beef mixture. Repeat this for the remaining waffles, broil for around 1-2 minutes until the cheese has melted then serve right away.

Nutrition:

- 18.8g Protein
- 33.9g Fats
- 415 Calories

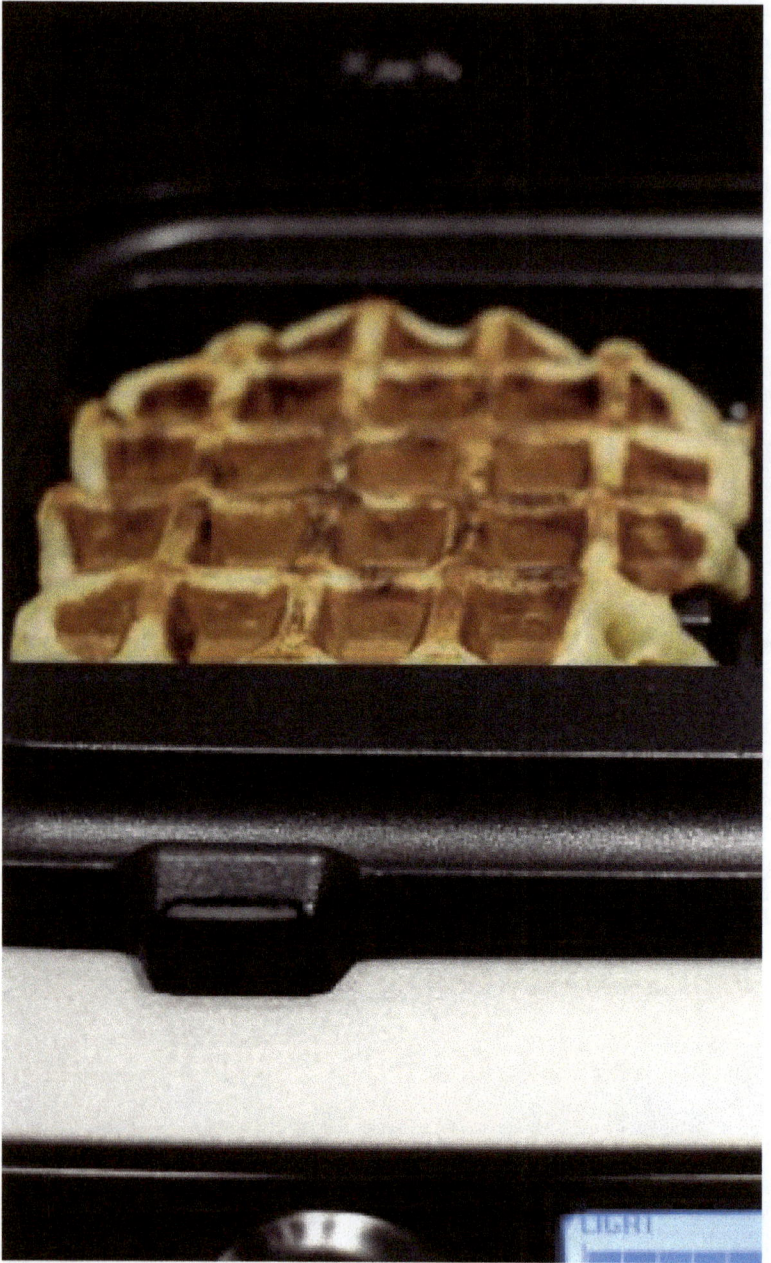

Keto Breakfast Cheesecake

Preparation Time: 20 minutes

Cooking Time: 45 minutes

Servings: 24

Ingredients:

Toppings:

- 1/4 cup of mixed berries for each cheesecake, frozen and thawed
- Filling ingredients
- 1/2 teaspoon of vanilla extract
- 1/2 teaspoon of almond extract
- 3/4 cup of sweetener
- 6 eggs
- 8 ounces of cream cheese
- 16 ounces of cottage cheese

Crust ingredients:

- 4 tablespoons of salted butter
- 2 tablespoons of sweetener
- 2 cups of almonds, whole

Direction:

1. Preheat oven to around 350 degrees F.

2. Pulse almonds in a food processor then add in butter and sweetener.

3. Pulse until all the ingredients mix well and coarse dough forms.

4. Coat twelve silicone muffin pans using foil or paper liners.

5. Portion the batter evenly between the muffin pans then press into the bottom part until it forms a crust and bakes for about 8 minutes.

6. Pulse in a food processor the cream cheese and cottage cheese then pulse until the mixture is smooth.

7. Put in the extracts and sweetener then combine until well mixed.

8. Add in eggs and pulse again until it becomes smooth. Share equally the batter between the muffin pans, then bake for around 30-40 minutes.

9. Put aside until cooled completely, then put in the refrigerator for about 2 hours and then top with frozen and thawed berries.

Nutrition:

- 12g Fats
- 152 Calories
- 6g Proteins

Egg-Crust Pizza

Preparation Time: 5 minutes

Cooking Time: 15 minutes Servings: 2

Ingredients:

- ¼ teaspoon of dried oregano to taste
- ½ teaspoon of spike seasoning to taste
- 1 ounce of mozzarella, chopped into small cubes
- 6 – 8 sliced thinly black olives
- 6 slices of turkey pepperoni, sliced into half
- 4-5 thinly sliced small grape tomatoes
- 2 eggs, beaten well
- 1-2 teaspoons of olive oil

Directions:

1. Preheat the broiler in an oven than in a small bowl, beat well the eggs. Cut the pepperoni and tomatoes in slices then cut the mozzarella cheese into cubes. Drizzle oil in a skillet at medium heat, then heat the pan for around one minute until it begins to get hot. Add in eggs and season with oregano and spike seasoning, then cook for around 2 minutes.

2. Drizzle half of the mozzarella, olives, pepperoni, and tomatoes on the eggs followed by another layer of the remaining half of the above ingredients. Ensure that

there is a lot of cheese on the topmost layers. Cover and cook for 4 minutes.

3. Position the pan under the preheated broiler and cook until the top has browned and the cheese has melted nicely for around 2-3 minutes. Serve immediately.

Nutrition

- 363 Calories
- 24.1g Fats
- 20.8g Carbohydrates

Breakfast Roll-Ups

Preparation Time: 5 minutes

Cooking Time: 15 minutes

Servings: 5

Ingredients:

- Non-stick cooking spray
- 5 patties of cooked breakfast sausage
- 5 slices of cooked bacon
- cups of cheddar cheese, shredded
- Pepper and salt
- 10 large eggs

Directions:

1. Prep a skillet on medium to high heat, then using a whisk, combine two of the eggs in a mixing bowl.
2. After the pan has become hot, lower the heat to medium-low heat then put in the eggs. If you want to, you can utilize some cooking spray.
3. Season eggs with some pepper and salt.
4. Seal the eggs and leave them to cook for a couple of minutes or until the eggs are almost cooked.
5. Drizzle around 1/3 cup of cheese on top of the eggs, then place a strip of bacon and divide the sausage into two and place on top.

6. Roll the egg carefully on top of the fillings. The roll-up will almost look like a taquitos. If you have a hard time folding over the egg, use a spatula to keep the egg intact until the egg has molded into a roll-up.

7. Put aside the roll-up then repeat the above steps until you have four more roll-ups; you should have 5 roll-ups in total.

Nutrition:

- 412.2g Calories
- 31.6g Fats
- 2.26g Carbohydrates

Basic Opie Rolls

Preparation Time: 20 minutes

Cooking Time: 35 minutes

Servings: 12

Ingredients:

- 1/8 teaspoon of salt
- 1/8 teaspoon of cream of tartar
- 3 ounces of cream cheese
- 3 large eggs

Direction:

1. Prepare oven to about 300 degrees, then separate the egg whites from egg yolks and place both eggs in different bowls. Using an electric mixer, beat well the egg whites until the mixture is very bubbly, then stir in the cream of tartar and mix.

2. In the bowl with the egg yolks, put in 3 ounces of cubed cheese and salt. Mix well until the mixture has doubled in size and is pale yellow. Put in the egg white mixture into the egg yolk mixture then fold the mixture gently together.

3. Spray some oil on the cookie sheet coated with some parchment paper, then add dollops of the batter and bake for around 30 minutes.

4. You will know they are ready when the upper part of the rolls is firm and golden. Put aside on a wire rack. Enjoy with some coffee.

Nutrition:

- 45 Calories
- 4g Fats
- 2g Proteins

Almond Coconut Egg Wraps

Preparation time: 5 minutes

Cooking time: 5 minutes

Servings: 4

Ingredients:

- 5 Organic eggs
- 1 tbsp. Coconut flour
- 25 tsp. Sea salt
- 2 tbsp. almond meal

Directions:

1. Combine the fixings in a blender and work them until creamy. Heat a skillet using the med-high temperature setting.
2. Fill two tablespoons of batter into the skillet and cook - covered about three minutes. Turn it over to cook for another 3 minutes. Serve the wraps piping hot.

Nutrition:

- 3g Carbohydrates
- 8g Protein
- 111 Calories

Bacon & Avocado Omelet

Preparation Time: 5 minutes

Cooking Time: 5 minutes

Servings: 1

Ingredients:

- 1 slice Crispy bacon
- 2 Large organic eggs
- 5 cup freshly grated parmesan cheese
- 2 tbsp. Ghee or coconut oil or butter
- half of 1 small Avocado

Directions:

1. Prepare the bacon to your liking and set aside. Combine the eggs, parmesan cheese, and your choice of finely chopped herbs. Warm a skillet and add the butter/ghee to melt using the medium-high heat setting. When the pan is hot, whisk and add the eggs.
2. Prepare the omelet working it towards the middle of the pan for about 30 seconds. When firm, flip, and cook it for another 30 seconds.
3. Arrange the omelet on a plate and garnish with the crunched bacon bits. Serve with sliced avocado.

Nutrition:

- 3.3g Carbohydrates
- 30g Protein
- 719 Calories

Bacon & Cheese Frittata

Preparation Time: 5 minutes

Cooking Time: 5 minutes

Servings: 6

Ingredients:

- 1 cup Heavy cream
- 6 Eggs
- 5 Crispy slices of bacon
- 2 Chopped green onions
- 4 oz. Cheddar cheese

Directions:

1. Warm the oven temperature to reach 350° Fahrenheit.
2. Scourge eggs and seasonings. Fill into the pie pan and top off with the remainder of the fixings. Bake 30-35 minutes. Wait for a few minutes before serving for best results.

Nutrition:

- 2g Carbohydrates
- 13g Protein
- 320 Calories

Bacon & Egg Breakfast Muffins

Preparation Time: 15 minutes

Cooking Time: 30 minutes

Servings: 12

Ingredients:

- 8 large Eggs
- 8 slices Bacon
- .66 cup Green onion

Directions:

1. Warm the oven at 350° Fahrenheit. Spritz the muffin tin wells using a cooking oil spray. Chop the onions and set aside.

2. Prepare a large skillet using the medium temperature setting. Fry the bacon until it's crispy and place on a layer of paper towels to drain the grease. Chop it into small pieces after it has cooled.

3. Whisk the eggs, bacon, and green onions, mixing well until all of the fixings are incorporated. Dump the egg mixture into the muffin tin (halfway full). Bake it for about 20 to 25 minutes. Cool slightly and serve.

Nutrition:

- 0.4g Carbohydrates

- 5.6g Protein
- 69 Calories

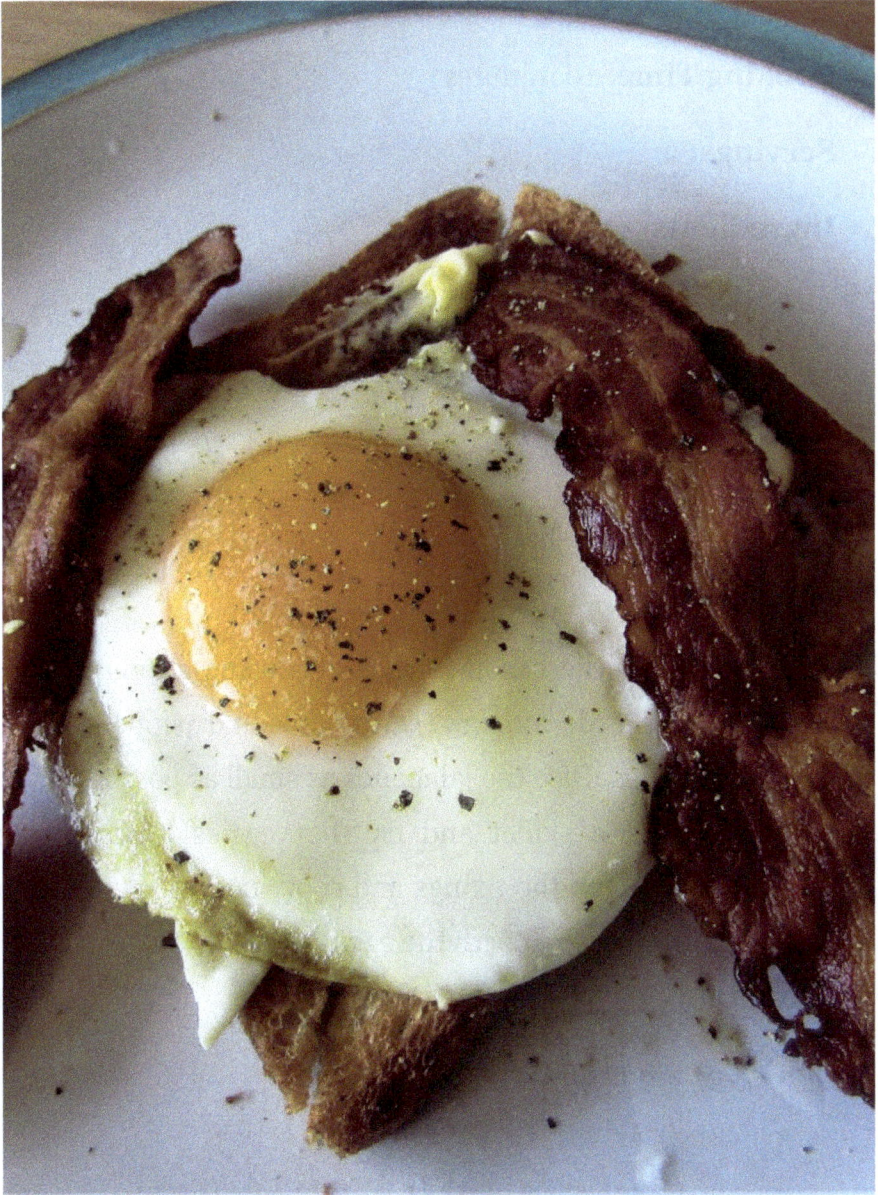

Bacon Hash

Preparation Time: 5 minutes

Cooking Time: 10 minutes

Servings: 2

Ingredients:

- 1 Small green pepper
- 2 Jalapenos
- 1 Small onion
- 4 Eggs
- 6 Bacon slices

Directions:

1. Chop the bacon into chunks using a food processor. Set aside for now. Cut onions and peppers into thin strips. Dice the jalapenos as small as possible.
2. Heat a skillet and fry the veggies. Once browned, combine the fixings and cook until crispy. Place on a serving dish with the eggs.

Nutrition:

- 9g Carbohydrates
- 23g Protein
- 366 Calories

Keto Peanut Butter Bars

Preparation Time: 5 minutes

Cooking Time: 15 minutes

Serving: 10

Ingredients:

- Half a cup of coconut flour
- Two cups of smooth peanut butter
- Half cup of sweetener that is sticky

Directions:

1. Place a parchment paper in a square pan and line it with it
2. Put all the ingredients into a big mixing bowl and mix until it is fully combined
3. Pour the batter into the already lined baking pan and refrigerate it till it is firm.
4. When it is firm, cut it into 20 bars and serve.

Nutrition:

- 112 calories 8g Fat
- 4g Carbohydrates
- 4g Protein 3g Fiber

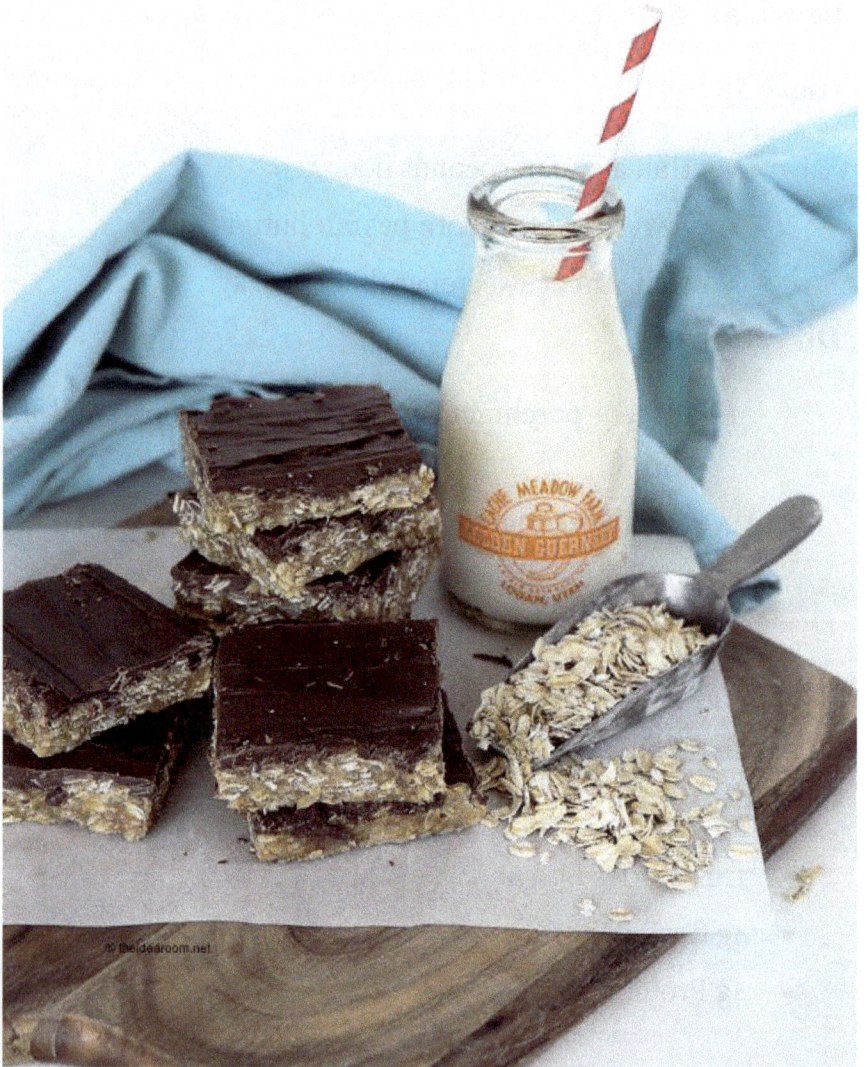

Keto Chocolate Crunch Bars

Preparation Time: 5 minutes

Cooking Time: 10 minutes

Serving: 10

Ingredients:

- One and a half cup of chocolate chips (of choice)
- One cup of almond butter (or any seed/nut butter of choice)
- A quarter cup of coconut oil
- Half cup of sweetener that is sticky
- Three cups of almond nuts or cashew nuts (or any other nuts you desire)

Directions:

1. Get a big baking dish and line it with parchment paper.
2. Get a bowl that is microwave friendly and mix the chocolate chips, the coconut oil, the almond butter and the sweetener and melt them till they combine.
3. Then add the almond nut or the cashew nut or your desired nuts and combine the mixture well by mixing it.
4. Pour the mixture into the already lined baking dish and let it spread.

5. Refrigerate the mixture till it is firm. When it is firm, cut it into 20 bars and serve.

Nutrition:

- 155 calories
- 12g Fat
- 4g Carbohydrate
- 7g Protein 2g Fiber

Keto Coconut Chocolate Bars

Preparation Time: 5 minutes

Cooking Time: 10 minutes

Serving: 10

Ingredients:

- Two cups of any type of chocolate chips desired
- One cup of coconut oil that is melted
- Three cups of coconut flakes that is shredded
- A quarter cup of sweetener

Directions:

1. Use a parchment paper to line the inside of a big baking pan. Get a big mixing bowl and put all of the ingredients. Mix the mixture to let it be well combined
2. Pour the batter (the mixture) in the already lined with parchment paper pan. Use your hands to press it firmly. Wet your hands to press it.
3. Refrigerate to make it firm. When it is firm, remove from the refrigerator, cut it into 20 bars, and put it back in the refrigerator.
4. Melt the chocolate chips and dip each of the coconut bars into the melted chocolate. Refrigerate again and serve.

Nutrition:

- 106 Calories
- 11g Total fat
- 3g Total carbohydrate
- 2g Protein

Keto Lemon Bars

Preparation Time: 30 minutes

Cooking Time: 15 minutes

Serving: 4

Ingredients:

- Three lemons
- One and a half cup of almond flour
- Half a cup of butter
- One cup of powdered sweetener

Directions:

1. Get a baking dish and line it with parchment paper. Mix a cup of the almond flour, a quarter of the sweetener, the butter and a pinch of salt in a medium mixing bowl. Pour this mixture into the baking dish that is already lined with parchment paper and bake for about 20 minutes. Remove and let it cool down.
2. Zest one of the lemons in a medium bowl and juice the three lemons. Put the eggs and the rest of the sweetener, the rest of the almond flour and add a pinch of salt. Mix to make the filling.
3. This filling can now be poured into the baked crust and bake for 15 minutes. Remove and serve with slices of lemon. Also sprinkle sweetener on it.

Nutrition:

- 193 calories
- 19 g Fat
- 4g Protein
- 3g Carbohydrates

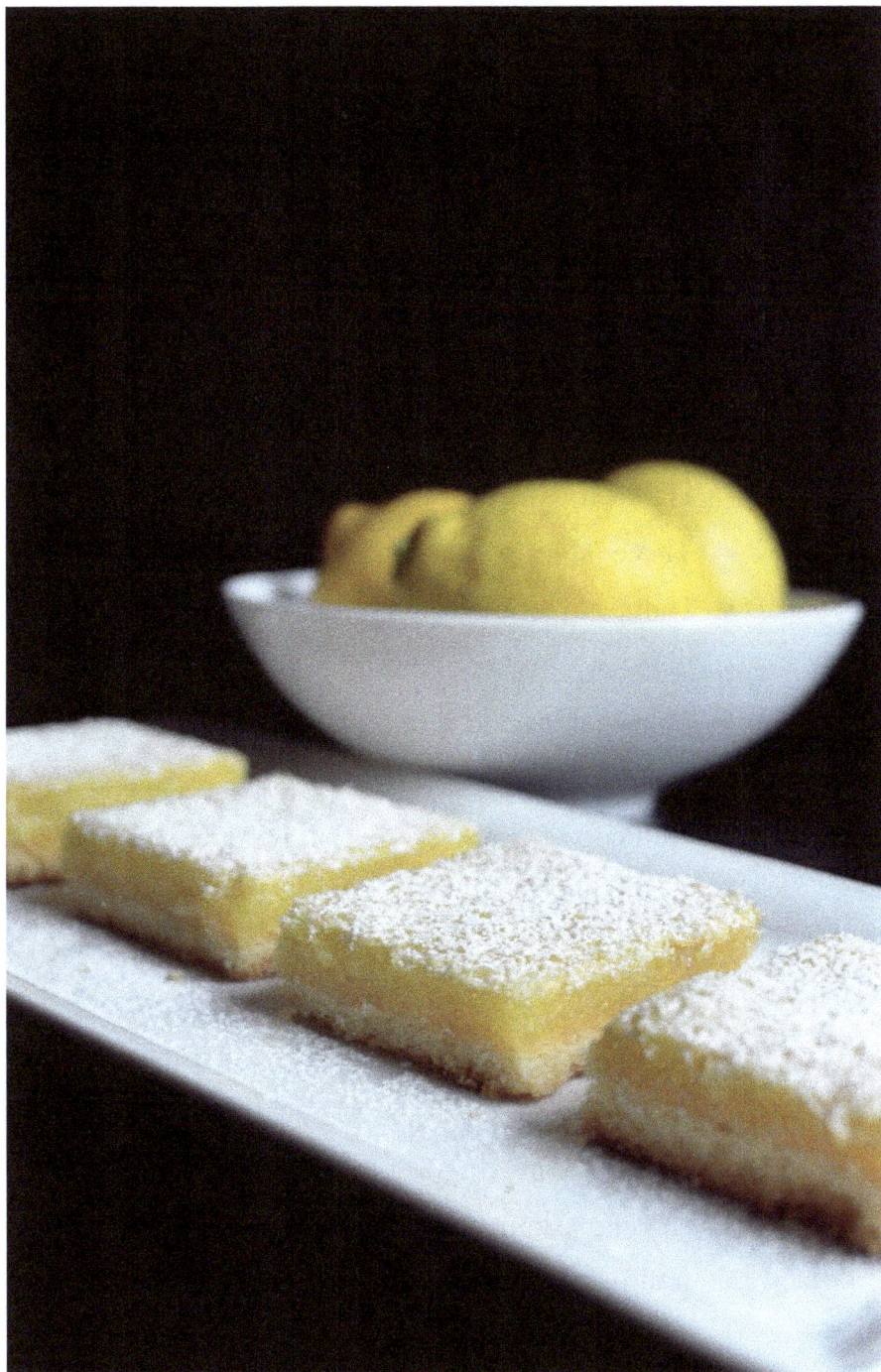

Chocolate Chip Pumpkin Protein Bar

Preparation Time: 5 minutes

Cooking Time: 10 minutes

Serving: 4

Ingredients:

- Two table spoons of chocolate chips that is sugar free
- Half a cup of coconut flour
- Three table spoons of protein powder
- Half a cup of pumpkin puree
- One table spoon of pumpkin pie spice
- Three table spoons of butter powder
- A pinch of salt
- Half cup of almond milk that is unsweetened
- Two table spoons of powdered sweetener

Directions:

1. Get a medium baking pan and line it with parchment paper Get a medium mixing bowl; add the butter powder flour, the protein powder, a pinch of salt, the coconut flour, the powdered sweetener and the pumpkin pie spice. Mix until they are well combined.

2. Add the pumpkin puree and the almond milk and stir well until they have combined well. Also add the chocolate chips and stir.
3. Pour the mixture into the baking pan and make it firm by pressing it down. Refrigerate for some minutes and slice in to bars, then serve.

Nutrition:

- 89.1 Calories
- 2.7g Fat
- 7.1g Protein
- 5.7g Carbohydrate

Keto Flourless Chocolate Cake

Preparation Time: 10 minutes

Cooking Time: 30 minutes

Serving: 4

Ingredients:

- One and a half cup of cocoa powder
- Two table spoons of baking powder
- Two and a half spoons of Dutch cocoa
- One and a half cup of milk (use a plant-based milk like coconut milk, almond milk or other plant-based milk of choice for the vegan version of the keto flourless chocolate cake)
- One and a half table spoon of flavor of choice
- One cup of sugar (coconut sugar or date sugar of half of a cup of erythritol for the gluten free version)

Directions:

1. First of all, heat the oven to about 350°F Get a baking pan and line it with the parchment paper
2. In a big mixing bowl, mix all the dry ingredients (the cocoa powder, the Dutch cocoa, the baking powder, the coconut sugar or the date sugar Use a mixer to whisk the eggs. Do this till the size has doubled and till it is frothy.

3. In another small mixing bowl, mix the wet ingredients (the milk and the flavor) gently add the mixed wet ingredients to the mixed dry ingredients and stir.

4. Pour the mixture into the already lined baking pan with parchment paper. Bake for about 30 minutes. Remove from baking pan and serve

Nutrition:

- 130 Calories
- 9g Total Fat
- 0.9g Saturated Fat
- 175mg Sodium

Brownie Cheese Cake

Preparation Time: 15 minutes

Cooking Time: 30 minutes

Serving: 4

Ingredients:

- Almond flour or coconut flour (that is finely ground)
- Butter (soft
- Erythritol (the powdered form)
- Cocoa powder: (Dutch baking cocoa powder)
- Vanilla extract (that is free of sugar)
- Cream cheese (the full fat type)
- Some chocolate bars (to be grated)

Directions:

1. For the brownie layer
2. Mix the Dutch baking cocoa powder and the vanilla extract in a mixing bowl until it has combined well add the soft butter and mix well. (be sure to make the butter mix well in the mixture to form a paste)
3. Pour the mixture (the brownie layer) halfway into an appropriate silicon mold of the desired size (be sure to fill it halfway to allow for the cheese layer also to be poured in it)

4. The brownie layer can be stored in a fridge pending the time the cheesecake layer would be ready.

5. For the cheese cake layer

6. Add the rest of the butter, the almond flour or coconut flour, the rest of the vanilla essence into a mixing bowl and mix till it is very smooth.

7. When it is very smooth, pour the mixture into the cooled half-filled silicon mold till it is filled up. Freeze in a freezer for about 2 hours or till it is hard enough. Remove the already made brownie cheesecake from the silicon mold carefully and serve.

Nutrition:

- 231 Calories
- 16.4g Total Fat
- 182mg Sodium
- 22.1g Total Carbohydrate

Peanut Butter Molten Lava Cake

Preparation Time: 25 minutes

Cooking Time: 15 minutes

Servings: 4

Ingredients:

- 2 huge eggs and their yolks
- A cup of peanut butter
- Chocolate sauce (that is low carb)
- Six full table spoons of almond flour
- one full table spoons of vanilla essence
- two table spoons of coconut oil
- seven tablespoons of sweetener (powered form)
- a spoon of butter to grease the baking pan

Directions:

1. Heat the oven to about 370F. Use the butter to grease the baking pan very well so that the cake would remove smoothly without any dent.

2. Put the coconut oil and peanut butter into a bowl that is microwave safe and stir. Heat them for a little while to get it melted. When the mixture is already melted, stir it well till it mixes and is smooth.

3. Add the powdered sweetener into the melted mixture and whisk it. Also add the almond flour, the vanilla

essence, the eggs and their yolks. Shake and mix the mixture until it is very smooth.

4. Fill the baking pan with the swap and bake for about 15 minutes. Once done, remove the cake from the pan using a knife to loosen the cake from the baking pan.

5. Place on a serving plate and drizzle it with the chocolate sauce (that is low in carbohydrate) Follow this process for the four cakes

Nutrition:

- 387 Calories
- 35.02g Total Fat
- 10.44g Protein
- 6.41g Carbohydrate
- 1.13g Fiber

Chocolate Japanese Cheesecake

Preparation Time: 20 minutes

Cooking Time: 40 minutes

Servings: 8

Ingredients:

- 3 pieces egg
- 120 g Cream Cheese (Philadelphia)
- 100g Sugar Free Chocolate
- ½ tsp. Lemon juice

Directions:

1. Preheat your oven to 170 ° C (top and bottom heat, without convection) and place a pan with water on the bottom. Cover the bottom and sides of the 20 cm baking dish with parchment and grease it with oil; Wrap foil outside.
2. Separate the whites from the yolks. Beat the proteins at low speed until foam; add lemon juice and beat at high speed until steady peaks.
3. Melt your chocolate in water bath, add cream cheese to it and mix until smooth. Remove from heat, cool slightly, add yolks and mix thoroughly.

4. Gently add the proteins to the chocolate mixture (one-third at a time), mix and pour the dough into a baking dish.

5. Place the pan directly on a baking sheet with water and cook for 15 minutes. Then lower the temperature to 150 ° C and cook for another 20 minutes. Turn off the oven and leave the cheesecake in it for another 20 minutes.

Nutrition:

- 135 Calories 11g Fat
- 6g Carbohydrate
- 4g Fiber
- 4g Protein

Italian Cream Cake

Preparation Time: 30 minutes

Cooking Time: 1 hour

Servings: 4

Ingredients:

For the Cake:

- Two cups of almond flour
- One cup of coconut flour
- One cup of softened butter that is unsalted
- 4 huge eggs
- 1 cup of erythritol
- A pinch of salt
- 2 table spoon of baking powder
- One cup of heavy cream
- Half table spoon of cream of tartar
- One table spoon of vanilla extract
- One cup of pecans (already chopped)
- One cup of already shredded coconut

For the frosting:

- Half cup of heavy cream
- One cup of soft butter that is unsalted
- Two table spoons of vanilla extract

- One cup of cream cheese
- Half cup of swerve (powdered)
- For the garnish
- Two table spoons of pecans that are chopped already
- Two table spoons of shredded coconut that are toasted

Directions:

1. Before starting the preparation, first heat the oven to about 350F. Use the parchment paper lining to line the inside of the cake baking pan and grease it with a little butter for easy remover

2. Add the flour, the baking powder, the salt and the pecans and coconut into a large bowl and stir. In another bowl, put the sweetener and the butter and cream it until it becomes very fluffy and light.

3. Remove the yolks from the egg and beat them. Then add to the mixture of sweetener and butter and mix it well. Then add the heavy cream and the vanilla to the above mixture and mix it very well again.

4. Add the dry ingredients (the almond flour, the coconut flour, the salt and the baking powder) in to the mixed butter mixture and stir until it is fully combined. Put the egg whites of the already removed yolk into a bowl and whisk it together with the cream of tartar. Mix it well until it foams.

5. Then fold this mixture into the already mixed barter. To make the batter light, be sure to fold the egg white mixture lightly.

6. Pour the battered mixture into the baking pan and allow it to bake for about 40 minutes in the already heated oven. By this time, the edges of the cake should be a shade of golden brown and the center of the cake should be firm.

7. Leave it in the baking pans to cool. Remove the cake from the pans when they are already cool.

8. For the frosting

9. Put the cream cheese and the butter together in a mixing bowl and start to mix them until the mixture becomes very fluffy and light.

10. To the mixture, add the sweetener and the vanilla and mix it by beating the mixture.

11. Next, add the heavy cream to the mixture. To get your desired consistency, add the heavy cream slowly so as to be able to stop when it reaches the desired consistency.

12. Paste the top of the cake and the side of the cake with the frosting.

13. On the top layer of the cake, sprinkle the roasted coconut that was shredded and use to decorate the cake.

Nutrition:

- 40g Carbohydrates
- 0g Dietary Fiber
- 28g Sugar
- 30g Fat

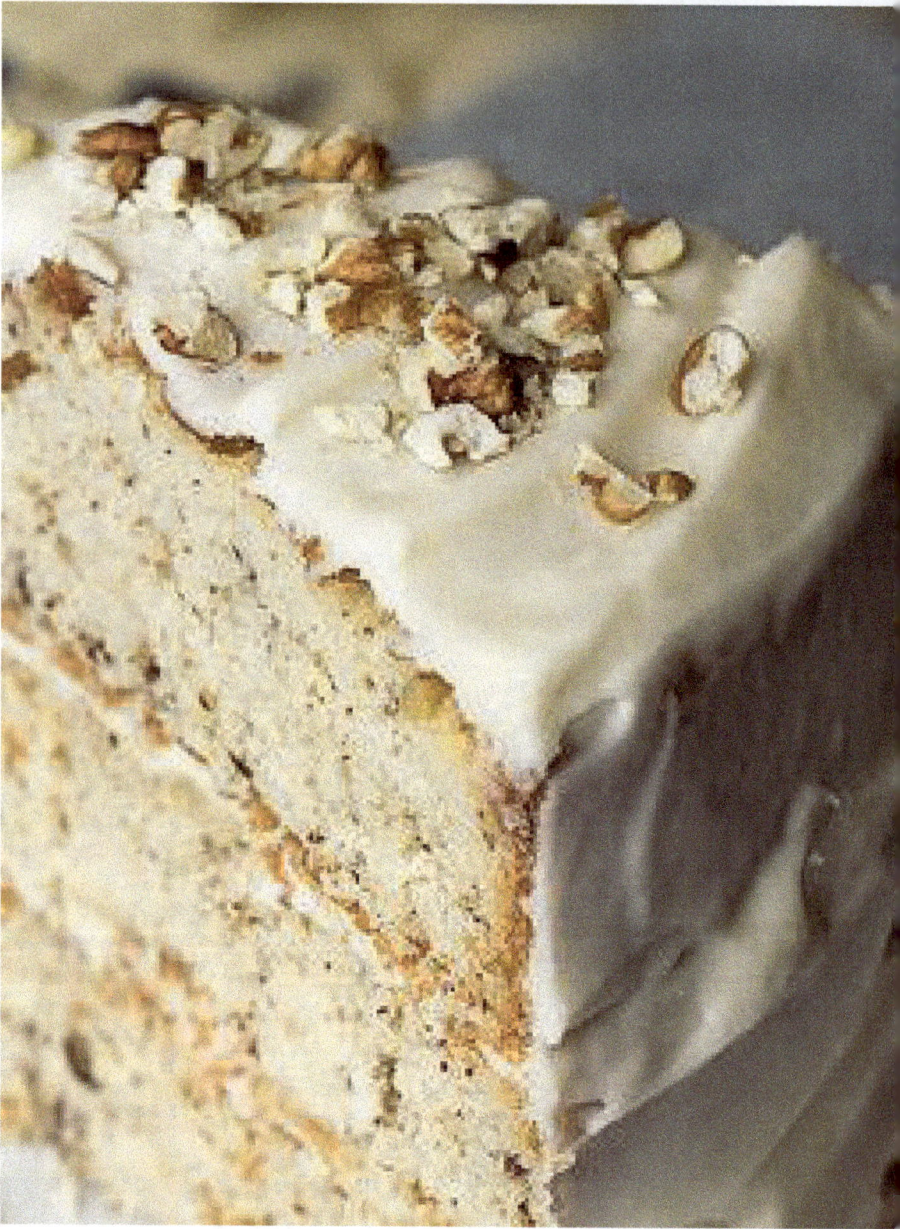

www.ingramcontent.com/pod-product-compliance
Lightning Source LLC
Chambersburg PA
CBHW050751030426
42336CB00012B/1768